INTRODUCTION : SETTING THE STAGE FOR OPTIMAL HEALTH, WEALTH, AND WELL-BEING

Welcome to a journey of self-discovery and personal growth that will empower you to thrive in all aspects of your life. This book is about setting the stage for optimal health, wealth, and well-being, and creating a life that is fulfilling, purpose-driven, and abundant.

In today's fast-paced and competitive world, it's easy to get caught up in the pursuit of external success, such as wealth, power, and recognition. However, true success is much more than just material possessions; it's about finding balance and harmony in all areas of your life, including your physical health, mental and emotional well-being, relationships, and finances.

The connection between health, wealth, and well-being is intricately intertwined. Your physical health affects your mental and emotional well-being, and your financial well-being impacts your overall quality of life. Thriving in all these areas requires intentional and mindful efforts, and this book will guide you on this journey.

Through practical strategies, insightful anecdotes, and evidence-based research, we will explore the key elements of optimal health, wealth, and well-being. We will discuss the importance of taking care of your physical health through proper nutrition, regular exercise, and self-care practices. We will delve into the realm of financial literacy and discuss strategies for managing your finances wisely, creating wealth, and achieving financial security. We will also delve into the realm of well-being, including the importance of mental, emotional, and spiritual health, and how they impact your overall well-being and success in life.

But this book is not just about external strategies and tactics; it's also about inner growth and self-awareness. We will emphasize the importance of self-reflection, self-awareness, and continuous personal growth as essential elements of your journey to optimal health, wealth, and well-being. Understanding your values, beliefs, strengths, and weaknesses, and aligning them with your goals and aspirations, will be a key focus of our exploration.

We will also recognize that setbacks and failures are inevitable in life, but they can serve as valuable learning opportunities. Embracing failure as a stepping stone to success, rather than a roadblock, will be an important mindset to cultivate on this journey. We will also explore the power of resilience, perseverance, and mindset in overcoming challenges and achieving long-term success.

The journey to optimal health, wealth, and well-being is not a one-size-fits-all approach. It's a unique and individual path that requires self-awareness, intentional action, and a commitment to continuous growth. This book will serve as your guide, providing you with the tools, insights, and inspiration to create a life that is aligned with your values, beliefs, and aspirations.

So, are you ready to set the stage for optimal health, wealth, and

Table of Contents:

Introduction: Setting the Stage for Optimal Health, Wealth, and Well-Being

Chapter 1: The Foundation of Health, Wealth, and Well-Being

Chapter 2: Nurturing Your Physical Health

Chapter 3: Cultivating Mental and Emotional Wellness

Chapter 4: The Power of Financial Literacy

Chapter 5: Building a Wealth Mindset

Chapter 6: Creating and Managing Wealth

Chapter 7: The Art of Work-Life Balance

Chapter 8: Cultivating Meaningful Relationships

Chapter 9: The Science of Happiness

Chapter 10: Embracing Change and Resilience

Chapter 11: Living with Purpose and Passion

Chapter 12: Creating a Lasting Legacy

Conclusion: Thriving in Health, Wealth, and Well-Being: Your Journey to Success

well-being in your life? Are you ready to embark on a journey of self-discovery and personal growth that will empower you to thrive in all areas of your life? If so, let's dive in and begin this transformative journey together. May you find abundance, joy, and fulfillment in all aspects of your life, and may this book be a beacon of guidance and inspiration on your path to optimal health, wealth, and well-being.

CHAPTER 1: THE FOUNDATION OF HEALTH, WEALTH, AND WELL-BEING

The pursuit of a fulfilling and successful life encompasses more than just one aspect. It involves the interconnectedness of multiple facets, including health, wealth, and well-being. In this chapter, we will lay the foundation for understanding the crucial role that optimal health, abundant wealth, and overall well-being play in achieving a harmonious and prosperous life.

The Importance of Health in Achieving Success. Good health is the cornerstone of a fulfilling life. Without robust physical and mental health, it becomes challenging to pursue our goals and aspirations effectively. Optimal health not only empowers us to perform at our best but also enhances our overall well-being and quality of life.

Maintaining physical health involves various aspects, including regular exercise, proper nutrition, sufficient sleep, and stress management. Regular exercise helps to keep our bodies strong, improves cardiovascular health, and enhances cognitive function. Proper nutrition provides our bodies with the necessary nutrients for optimal functioning, while sufficient sleep allows for proper rest and recovery. Managing stress is crucial in maintaining good mental health, as excessive stress can negatively impact our physical and mental well-being.

In addition to physical health, mental health plays a vital role in our overall well-being. Mental health encompasses our emotional, psychological, and social well-being. It affects how we think, feel, and act, and impacts our relationships and daily functioning. Taking care of our mental health involves strategies such as self-care, stress management techniques, seeking professional help when needed, and maintaining healthy social connections.

In the pursuit of success, it's important to prioritize our health and well-being. When we are in good health, we have the energy, focus, and resilience to overcome challenges, pursue opportunities, and achieve our goals.

The Role of Wealth in Enabling Opportunities. Wealth, or financial well-being, is another critical aspect of a fulfilling life. It provides us with the resources and opportunities to pursue our passions, invest in ourselves and our future, and create a comfortable lifestyle for ourselves and our loved ones.

Building wealth requires smart financial management, including budgeting, saving, investing, and minimizing debt. It's crucial to have a clear understanding of our financial goals, create a plan to achieve them, and consistently take steps towards their attainment. This may involve developing financial literacy, seeking advice from financial professionals, and making informed decisions about spending, saving, and investing.

Wealth also provides us with the ability to seize opportunities and take calculated risks. It allows us to invest in education, acquire new skills, start a business, or pursue our passions without being limited by financial constraints. Having financial security provides peace of mind and reduces stress, allowing us to focus on our personal and professional growth.

Moreover, wealth can also be used for giving back and making a positive impact on our communities and the world. Philanthropy and charitable giving are ways to use wealth for the greater good, contributing to the well-being of others and making a meaningful difference in the lives of those in need.

The Interconnectedness of Health, Wealth, and Well-Being. Health and wealth are not isolated aspects of our lives but are deeply interconnected. They influence and impact each other in various ways, and both are essential for overall well-being and success.

For instance, good health is a critical foundation for building wealth. When we are in good health, we have the physical and mental capacity to pursue opportunities, work effectively, and make informed decisions. Optimal health also reduces the risk of health-related expenses, such as medical bills and lost productivity, which can impact our financial stability.

On the other hand, wealth can also positively impact our health and well-being. It provides us with the resources to invest in our health, such as accessing quality healthcare, purchasing nutritious food, and engaging in physical activities or fitness programs. Financial stability also reduces stress related to financial concerns, which can have a significant impact on our mental health and overall well-being.

Furthermore, well-being encompasses not only physical and financial health but also emotional, social, and spiritual well-being. These aspects are interconnected and mutually influence each other. For example, strong social connections and supportive relationships can positively impact our mental health and overall well-being. Engaging in activities that bring joy, fulfillment, and purpose can also contribute to our overall sense of well-being, which in turn can enhance our physical and mental health.

In summary, health, wealth, and well-being are interconnected and form the foundation of a fulfilling and successful life. They are interdependent and mutually influence each other, and neglecting one aspect can impact the others. Therefore, it's essential to prioritize and invest in our health, wealth, and well-being holistically, recognizing their interconnections and their crucial role in achieving a balanced and prosperous life.

In conclusion, mastering the art of optimal health, wealth, and well-being is vital for achieving a fulfilling and successful life. This chapter has laid the foundation for understanding the importance of health, wealth, and well-being and their interconnections. We have explored how good health provides the physical and mental capacity to pursue opportunities, how wealth enables us to invest in ourselves and our future, and how well-being encompasses various aspects of our lives.

By recognizing the interconnectedness of health, wealth, and well-being and prioritizing them holistically, we can create a strong foundation for our personal and professional success. It's important to adopt healthy lifestyle practices, manage our finances wisely, and cultivate a sense of well-being that encompasses physical, mental, emotional, social, and spiritual aspects of our lives.

In the subsequent chapters of this book, we will delve deeper into each of these aspects and explore practical strategies and techniques for mastering the art of optimal health, wealth, and well-being. With the right mindset, knowledge, and actions, we can create a harmonious and prosperous life that brings us joy, fulfillment, and success.

CHAPTER 2: NURTURING YOUR PHYSICAL HEALTH

Physical health is the foundation of overall well-being. It provides us with the energy, vitality, and resilience to lead a fulfilling life. Nurturing our physical health involves adopting healthy lifestyle practices, such as maintaining a balanced diet, engaging in regular exercise, getting enough sleep, and managing stress. In this chapter, we will delve into the importance of physical health and explore practical strategies and techniques for nurturing it.

The Importance of a Healthy Diet. A healthy diet plays a crucial role in maintaining optimal physical health. It provides the nutrients our bodies need to function properly and supports our immune system, which plays a critical role in protecting us from diseases and infections. In this section, we will discuss the importance of a well-balanced diet that includes a variety of foods from different food groups, such as fruits, vegetables, whole grains, lean proteins, and healthy fats. We will also explore the impact of poor dietary habits, such as excessive sugar, salt, and unhealthy fats consumption, on our physical health, and discuss practical tips for making healthier food choices.

The Benefits of Regular Exercise. Regular exercise is a key component of maintaining good physical health. It helps us build strength, endurance, and flexibility, improves our cardiovascular health, and supports weight management. Exercise also has numerous mental health benefits, such as reducing stress, improving mood, and boosting cognitive function. In this section, we will explore the benefits of regular exercise for our physical and mental health and discuss different types of exercises, such as aerobic exercises, strength training, and flexibility exercises, and how to incorporate them into our daily routine. We will also discuss strategies for overcoming barriers to exercise, such as lack of time or motivation, and provide practical tips for establishing a sustainable exercise routine.

The Importance of Adequate Sleep. Sleep is a fundamental aspect of physical health and well-being. It plays a crucial role in rest and recovery, allowing our bodies to repair and rejuvenate. Poor sleep quality or inadequate sleep duration can have detrimental effects on our physical health, including increased risk of chronic conditions such as obesity, diabetes, cardiovascular diseases, and impaired immune function. In this section, we will discuss the importance of adequate sleep for our physical health, explore the factors that influence sleep quality and duration, and provide practical tips for improving our sleep hygiene.

Managing Stress for Physical Health. Stress can have a significant impact on our physical health. Chronic stress can lead to a variety of health issues, such as high blood pressure, weakened immune system, and increased risk of chronic diseases. Therefore, it's essential to manage stress effectively for optimal physical health. In this section, we will discuss the impact of stress on our physical health, explore different stress management techniques, such as mindfulness, relaxation techniques, and time management, and provide practical tips for reducing and managing stress in our daily lives.

Nurturing our physical health is fundamental to our overall well-being. Adopting healthy lifestyle practices, such as maintaining a balanced diet, engaging in regular exercise, getting enough sleep, and managing stress, are crucial for optimal physical health. By prioritizing and incorporating these practices into our daily lives, we can lay a strong foundation for our physical well-being and enhance our overall quality of life. In the subsequent chapters, we will continue to explore other aspects of health, wealth, and well-being, and provide practical strategies for mastering the art of optimal living.

CHAPTER 3: CULTIVATING MENTAL AND EMOTIONAL WELLNESS

Mental and emotional wellness are integral components of overall well-being. Our mental and emotional health greatly impact our thoughts, feelings, behaviors, and quality of life. Cultivating mental and emotional wellness involves developing healthy coping strategies, managing stress, building resilience, and fostering positive emotional states. In this chapter, we will explore the importance of mental and emotional wellness, and provide practical strategies and techniques for nurturing them.

Understanding Mental Health. Mental health refers to our psychological and emotional well-being. It encompasses our thoughts, feelings, and behaviors, and how we cope with stress, challenges, and life events. Understanding mental health is crucial for cultivating optimal mental well-being. In this section, we will discuss the importance of mental health, common misconceptions and stigmas associated with mental health, and the impact of mental health on our overall well-being. We will also explore the signs and symptoms of common mental health conditions, such as anxiety, depression, and stress, and discuss strategies for seeking professional help when needed.

Building Emotional Intelligence. Emotional intelligence is the ability to recognize, understand, and manage our own emotions and the emotions of others. It plays a vital role in our mental and emotional well-being, as it helps us navigate relationships, manage stress, and make healthy decisions. In this section, we will discuss the importance of emotional intelligence, explore the different components of emotional intelligence, such as self-awareness, self-regulation, empathy, and social skills, and provide practical tips for developing and enhancing our emotional intelligence.

Developing Healthy Coping Strategies. Healthy coping strategies are essential for managing stress, adversity, and challenges in life. They help us navigate difficult situations, regulate our emotions, and maintain mental and emotional wellness. In this section, we will discuss different healthy coping strategies, such as problem-solving, emotional regulation, positive reframing, and seeking social support. We will also explore the impact of unhealthy coping mechanisms, such as substance abuse, avoidance, and negative self-talk, on our mental and emotional health, and provide practical tips for developing healthy coping strategies.

Building Resilience. Resilience is the ability to bounce back from adversity and challenges, and maintain mental and emotional well-being. It is a crucial skill in navigating the ups and downs of life and managing stress and setbacks effectively. In this section, we will discuss the concept of resilience, explore the factors that contribute to resilience, such as social support, self-efficacy, and optimism, and provide practical strategies for building resilience, such as cultivating a growth mindset, developing problem-solving skills, and practicing self-compassion.

Cultivating mental and emotional wellness is crucial for our overall well-being. By understanding mental health, developing emotional intelligence, building healthy coping strategies, and fostering resilience, we can enhance our mental and emotional well-being and lead a more fulfilling life. In the subsequent chapters, we will continue to explore other aspects of health, wealth, and well-being, and provide practical strategies for mastering the art of optimal living.

CHAPTER 4: THE POWER OF FINANCIAL LITERACY

Financial literacy is a critical skill that plays a significant role in our overall well-being. It involves understanding and managing our personal finances effectively, including budgeting, saving, investing, and making informed financial decisions. Financial literacy empowers us to take control of our financial future, achieve financial goals, and build wealth for ourselves and our families. In this chapter, we will explore the importance of financial literacy, the impact of financial literacy on our financial well-being, and practical strategies for mastering the art of financial literacy.

Understanding the Basics of Personal Finance. To achieve financial literacy, it is essential to understand the basics of personal finance. In this section, we will discuss key concepts related to personal finance, such as budgeting, saving, investing, debt management, and credit management. We will explore the importance of budgeting as a foundation for managing our finances effectively, the benefits of saving and investing for long-term financial goals, strategies for managing debt responsibly, and the impact of credit management on our financial health. We will also provide practical tips and techniques for implementing these basic financial concepts into our daily lives.

Building Financial Knowledge and Skills. Building financial knowledge and skills is a crucial aspect of financial literacy. In this section, we will discuss strategies for expanding our financial knowledge and skills, including reading financial books and articles, taking financial courses, seeking advice from financial professionals, and staying informed about financial news and trends. We will also explore the importance of understanding financial products and services, such as savings accounts, retirement accounts, investment vehicles, insurance policies, and credit cards, and making informed decisions about them. Additionally, we will discuss the role of financial goal-setting, budgeting, and tracking expenses in building financial knowledge and skills.

Creating a Financial Plan. Creating a financial plan is a key step towards achieving financial literacy and success. In this section, we will discuss the importance of creating a comprehensive financial plan that aligns with our financial goals and values. We will explore the different components of a financial plan, such as setting short-term and long-term financial goals, creating a budget, establishing an emergency fund, developing a debt repayment strategy, and implementing an investment plan. We will also discuss the significance of regularly reviewing and updating our financial plan to adapt to changing circumstances and financial goals.

Managing Financial Risks. Managing financial risks is an essential aspect of financial literacy. In this section, we will discuss strategies for managing various financial risks, such as emergencies, unexpected expenses, job loss, disability, illness, and market fluctuations. We will explore the importance of having an emergency fund as a buffer for unexpected financial events, obtaining adequate insurance coverage, such as health insurance, disability insurance, and life insurance, and diversifying investments to minimize risk. We will also discuss the significance of regularly reviewing and updating our risk management strategies to protect our financial well-being.

Building Wealth and Investing. Building wealth and investing are critical components of financial literacy. In this section, we will discuss strategies for building wealth over the long term, such as investing in stocks, bonds, real estate, and other investment vehicles. We will explore the importance of diversification, asset allocation, and risk tolerance in investment decisions, as well as the significance of long-term investing and compounding. We will also discuss the role of financial advisors, the impact of fees and expenses on investment returns, and the importance of regularly reviewing and rebalancing investment portfolios to achieve financial goals.

In conclusion, financial literacy is a powerful tool that empowers us to take control of our financial future and achieve

CHAPTER 5: BUILDING A WEALTH MINDSET

Building wealth is not just about accumulating money; it's also about developing the right mindset to manage and grow your financial resources. Your mindset plays a critical role in your ability to create wealth and achieve financial success. In this chapter, we will explore the key elements of a wealth mindset and provide practical strategies to help you develop and cultivate it.

1. Embrace a Positive Money Mindset

One of the first steps in building a wealth mindset is to adopt a positive attitude towards money. Many people have negative beliefs about money that can hold them back from achieving financial success. For example, some may believe that money is evil, or that it's difficult to make money, or that rich people are greedy. These negative beliefs can create self-sabotaging behaviors and limit your ability to accumulate wealth.

To develop a positive money mindset, it's important to recognize and challenge these negative beliefs. Start by examining your own beliefs about money and identify any negative thought patterns that may be holding you back. Once you've identified them, replace them with positive affirmations and beliefs about money. For example, instead of believing that money is evil, you can choose to believe that money is a tool that can be used for good and to make a positive impact in the world.

It's also crucial to surround yourself with positive influences when it comes to money. Associate with people who have a positive money mindset and who can inspire and motivate you to achieve your financial goals. Avoid negative influences, such as people who constantly complain about money or who have a scarcity mentality. Surrounding yourself with positivity can help you shift your mindset and develop a more positive relationship with money.

2. Cultivate a Growth Mindset

A growth mindset is the belief that you can constantly learn, improve, and develop new skills. This mindset is essential for building wealth because it encourages you to embrace challenges, persevere through setbacks, and continuously learn and adapt to changing circumstances.

To cultivate a growth mindset, start by reframing your mindset towards failures and setbacks. Instead of seeing them as obstacles or reasons to give up, view them as opportunities to learn and grow. Embrace challenges and see them as opportunities to develop new skills and knowledge. When faced with setbacks, resist the urge to blame external factors and instead focus on what you can do differently to improve the situation.

It's also important to be open to learning and acquiring new skills. Continuously invest in yourself by learning from books, online courses, mentors, and other resources. Develop a curiosity to explore new areas of knowledge and acquire skills that can increase your earning potential and contribute to your wealth-building journey.

3. Practice Financial Discipline

Financial discipline is a critical element of a wealth mindset. It involves managing your money wisely, living below your means, and making intentional financial decisions that align with your long-term financial goals.

One key aspect of financial discipline is budgeting. Creating a budget allows you to track your expenses, understand your cash flow, and make informed decisions about how to allocate your resources. Start by creating a budget that reflects your financial goals, and track your expenses regularly to ensure that you are staying within your budget. Look for areas where you can cut expenses and save money, and be mindful of your spending habits.

Another important aspect of financial discipline is saving and investing. Saving money allows you to build an emergency fund for unexpected expenses and create a foundation for wealth-building. Aim to save at least 20% of your income and prioritize saving before spending. Consider automating your savings by setting up automatic transfers from your checking account to your savings or investment accounts.

Investing is also a key component of building wealth. Once you have established an emergency fund and paid off high-interest debt, start investing your savings in assets that can grow in value over time

CHAPTER 6: CREATING AND MANAGING WEALTH

Creating and managing wealth is a lifelong journey that requires careful planning, disciplined financial strategies, and a proactive approach to financial management. It is not just about accumulating money, but also about preserving and growing wealth to achieve your financial goals and ensure a secure future for yourself and your loved ones. In this chapter, we will explore key concepts and strategies for creating and managing wealth, including setting financial goals, developing a comprehensive financial plan, managing expenses, building a diversified investment portfolio, managing risk through diversification, and preserving wealth through estate planning, tax planning, philanthropy, and succession planning. We will also discuss the importance of seeking professional advice from financial experts to help you navigate the complexities of wealth management and make informed decisions.

Setting Financial Goals

The first step in creating and managing wealth is to set clear financial goals. Financial goals are specific targets that you want to achieve with your wealth, such as saving for retirement, buying a home, funding education, starting a business, or leaving a legacy for future generations. Setting financial goals provides a sense of direction and purpose for your financial decisions and helps you prioritize your spending, saving, and investment efforts. When setting financial goals, it's important to make them SMART - Specific, Measurable, Achievable, Relevant, and Time-bound. This means that your goals should be clear, quantifiable, realistic, aligned with your values and priorities, and have a timeline for completion. For example, instead of setting a vague goal like "save more money," a SMART financial goal would be "save $10,000 in a retirement account within the next 12 months."

Developing a Comprehensive Financial Plan

Once you have set your financial goals, the next step is to develop a comprehensive financial plan. A financial plan is a roadmap that outlines the strategies and actions you will take to achieve your financial goals. It includes an assessment of your current financial situation, a budget, a savings and investment plan, a risk management plan, a retirement plan, an estate plan, and a plan for achieving other financial goals. A comprehensive financial plan takes into account your income, expenses, debts, assets, investments, taxes, insurance coverage, and other financial factors to provide a holistic view of your financial situation and guide your financial decisions. It is important to regularly review and update your financial plan as your financial circumstances and goals evolve over time.

Managing Expenses

Effective expense management is a critical aspect of wealth creation and management. It involves understanding your spending patterns, tracking your expenses, and finding ways to optimize your spending to maximize savings and investments.

One key strategy for managing expenses is budgeting. A budget is a plan that outlines your income, expenses, and savings goals for a specific period, typically on a monthly or annual basis. Creating a budget helps you gain visibility into your spending habits, identify areas where you can cut back or optimize spending, and ensure that you are living within your means. It also allows you to allocate a portion of your income towards savings and investments, which are essential for building wealth over time. Another strategy for managing expenses is to practice mindful spending, which involves being conscious of your spending choices, avoiding unnecessary expenses, and prioritizing spending on essential needs and long-term financial goals.

Building a Diversified Investment Portfolio

Investing is a critical strategy for wealth creation and growth. By investing your money wisely, you can potentially earn returns that outpace inflation and build wealth over time. One key principle of investing is diversification, which involves spreading your investments across different asset classes, sectors, geographic regions, and investment vehicles to reduce risk and optimize returns. A diversified investment portfolio can help you weather market fluctuations and minimize the impact of any single investment on your overall portfolio.

Asset Allocation: Asset allocation involves dividing your investments among different asset classes, such as stocks, bonds, real estate, and cash, based on your risk tolerance, time horizon, and financial goals. It is a critical component of portfolio diversification as it helps to balance risk and potential returns. The right asset allocation strategy will depend on your individual financial situation, risk tolerance, and investment objectives. It's important to review and adjust your asset allocation periodically to ensure that it remains aligned with your changing financial circumstances and goals.

Investment Vehicles: There are various investment vehicles available for wealth creation, such as stocks, bonds, mutual funds, exchange-traded funds (ETFs), real estate, and alternative investments. Each investment vehicle has its own risks and potential returns, and it's important to understand them before making investment decisions. It's also essential to diversify your investments within each asset class to further spread risk. For example, within the stock market, diversifying across different industries and market caps can help reduce risk.

Risk Management: Managing risk is a critical aspect of wealth management. Risk refers to the potential for loss of value in investments or other assets. While investments offer the potential for higher returns, they also come with varying degrees of risk. It's important to understand and manage these risks to protect your wealth. One key strategy for managing risk is diversification, as mentioned earlier. By diversifying your investments, you can spread risk across different assets and reduce the impact of any single investment on your overall portfolio. It's also important to have an emergency fund to cover unexpected expenses and protect your investments from being prematurely liquidated during market downturns.

Tax Planning: Another important aspect of wealth management is tax planning. Taxes can significantly impact your wealth, and strategic tax planning can help you minimize your tax liabilities and optimize your overall financial plan. It's important to understand the tax implications of different investment vehicles and strategies, such as tax-deferred retirement accounts, capital gains, and dividend taxes. Consulting with a tax professional can help you navigate the complex tax landscape and develop tax-efficient strategies that align with your financial goals.

Estate Planning: Estate planning involves creating a plan for the transfer of your assets to your heirs or beneficiaries after your passing. It's important to have a well-thought-out estate plan to ensure that your wealth is transferred according to your wishes and to minimize estate taxes, probate costs, and potential family disputes. Estate planning involves creating a will, establishing trusts, designating beneficiaries for retirement accounts and insurance policies, and appointing guardians for minor children, among other considerations. It's important to work with an experienced estate planning attorney to develop a comprehensive estate plan that aligns with your financial goals and family dynamics.

Philanthropy: Philanthropy, or charitable giving, is another aspect of wealth management that allows you to make a positive impact on society while managing your wealth. Charitable giving can be an effective strategy for reducing your taxable income and estate tax liabilities, as well as leaving a legacy and supporting causes that are meaningful to you. There are various ways to incorporate philanthropy into your wealth management plan, such as establishing a donor-advised fund, creating a charitable trust, or making direct charitable gifts. It's important to work with a qualified financial advisor and tax professional to ensure that your philanthropic efforts align with your overall financial plan and tax strategies.

Succession Planning: If you have a family business or other assets that you plan to pass on to future generations, succession planning is crucial. Succession planning involves developing a plan for transferring ownership and management of your business or other assets to the next generation or other designated successors. It's important to have a well-structured succession plan in place to ensure a smooth transition and to minimize potential conflicts among family members or business partners. Succession planning may involve creating a family trust, setting up a buy-sell agreement, or establishing a clear process for selecting and grooming future leaders. It's important to start succession planning early and involve all relevant stakeholders to ensure a successful transition.

Insurance Planning: Insurance planning is an essential part of wealth management as it helps protect your wealth and mitigate potential risks. This may include life insurance, disability insurance, long-term care insurance, and liability insurance, among others. Insurance planning ensures that you and your family are financially protected in case of unexpected events such as illness, disability, or death. It's important to review your insurance needs periodically to ensure that they are adequate and aligned with your current financial situation and goals.

Monitoring and Review: Wealth management is an ongoing process that requires regular monitoring and review. It's important to review your financial plan, investment portfolio, and other wealth management strategies periodically to ensure that they are still aligned with your financial goals and objectives. Economic conditions, market trends, and personal circumstances may change over time, and adjustments may be needed to keep your wealth management plan on track. Regular communication and collaboration with your financial advisor, tax professional, and other relevant professionals can help ensure that your wealth management plan remains effective and responsive to changes in your financial situation.

Behavioral Finance: Understanding behavioral finance is also an important aspect of wealth management. Behavioral finance studies how human behavior and emotions influence financial decision-making. Emotions such as fear, greed, and overconfidence can impact investment decisions and potentially derail your wealth management plan. Being aware of your emotions and biases, and working with a qualified financial advisor who can provide objective guidance, can help you make rational and informed financial decisions that align with your long-term financial goals.

Creating and managing wealth requires careful planning, disciplined execution, and ongoing review and adjustment. It's important to develop a comprehensive wealth management plan that incorporates various aspects such as financial goal setting, budgeting, savings, investment management, risk management, tax planning, estate planning, philanthropy, succession planning, insurance planning, and behavioral finance. Working with qualified professionals such as financial advisors, tax professionals, estate planning attorneys, and insurance agents can help you develop a customized wealth management plan that aligns with your individual financial situation, goals, and values.

Remember that wealth creation is a long-term endeavor that requires patience, discipline, and sound financial strategies. It's important to regularly review and adjust your wealth management plan as your financial circumstances and goals evolve. With careful planning and prudent management, you can create and manage wealth to achieve your financial goals, protect your assets, and leave a lasting legacy for future generations.

CHAPTER 7: THE ART OF WORK-LIFE BALANCE

As the demands of modern life continue to increase, finding balance between work and personal life has become a significant challenge for many individuals. Long working hours, increased workloads, and the constant connectivity of technology have blurred the boundaries between work and personal time, making it difficult to maintain a healthy work-life balance. However, achieving this balance is crucial for our overall well-being and happiness. In this chapter, we will explore the art of work-life balance and provide practical strategies for creating a fulfilling and harmonious life that encompasses both work and personal pursuits.

Understanding Work-Life Balance

Work-life balance refers to the equilibrium between the time and energy dedicated to work and the time and energy dedicated to personal life, including family, relationships, health, hobbies, and self-care. It involves finding a healthy integration of these two aspects of life so that they complement and support each other, rather than competing against each other.

Achieving work-life balance is a highly individualized process, as different people have different priorities, values, and commitments. What might be a balanced work-life arrangement for one person may not be the same for another. It is important to recognize that work-life balance is not a one-size-fits-all concept, and it may evolve and change over time as personal circumstances and priorities shift.

The Benefits of Work-Life Balance

Maintaining a healthy work-life balance has numerous benefits that positively impact both our personal and professional lives. Some of the key benefits of work-life balance include:

1. Enhanced well-being: A balanced approach to work and personal life can improve our physical and mental well-being. It allows us to manage stress, reduce the risk of burnout, and maintain good health, which in turn positively affects our overall quality of life.

2. Increased productivity: When we are well-rested, mentally and physically healthy, and emotionally fulfilled, we are more likely to be productive and efficient in our work. Balancing work with personal activities helps us to recharge and refocus, leading to increased creativity, motivation, and job satisfaction.

3. Improved relationships: Work-life balance enables us to devote time and attention to our personal relationships, including family, friends, and partners. This strengthens our connections and fosters positive relationships, which are crucial for our emotional well-being and social support system.

4. Greater happiness: Achieving a healthy work-life balance allows us to pursue our personal passions, hobbies, and interests, which bring joy and fulfillment to our lives. When we have a sense of purpose and meaning beyond work, it leads to greater life satisfaction and happiness.

Strategies for Achieving Work-Life Balance

While achieving work-life balance may seem challenging, there are several practical strategies that can help individuals create a balanced and fulfilling life. Here are some strategies to consider:

1. Define your priorities: Begin by identifying your values and priorities in both work and personal life. What matters most to you? What are your long-term goals? Understanding your priorities will help you make informed decisions and allocate your time and energy accordingly.

2. Set clear boundaries: Establish clear boundaries between work and personal time. Avoid checking work emails or engaging in work-related activities during personal time. Communicate your boundaries with your employer, colleagues, and family members, and stick to them as much as possible.

3. Plan and organize: Plan and organize your time effectively to ensure that you have dedicated time for work, personal commitments, and self-care. Create a schedule or a to-do list that includes both work and personal tasks, and prioritize them based on your values and goals.

4. Practice self-care: Make self-care a priority in your life. Take care of your physical, mental, and emotional well-being by getting regular exercise, eating healthy, getting enough sleep, and engaging in activities that bring you joy and relaxation. Make sure to also set aside time for hobbies, leisure activities, and spending time with loved ones.

5. Learn to say no: It's important to set boundaries and learn to say no when necessary. Avoid overcommitting yourself to work or personal activities that may disrupt your work-life balance. Be assertive in communicating your limitations and be willing to decline tasks or invitations that may overwhelm you.

6. Delegate and prioritize: Learn to delegate tasks at work and at home to ease your workload and free up time for personal activities. Prioritize your tasks based on their importance and urgency, and focus on completing the most critical tasks first. This will help you manage your time more effectively and avoid feeling overwhelmed.

7. Unplug from technology: Constant connectivity to technology can blur the boundaries between work and personal life. Practice unplugging from technology during your personal time to be fully present and engaged in your personal activities. Avoid checking work emails or engaging in work-related tasks during your personal time to create a clear separation between work and personal life.

8. Communicate with your employer: Open and honest communication with your employer is crucial in achieving work-life balance. Discuss your work expectations, workload, and any concerns or challenges you may be facing in balancing work and personal life. Work together with your employer to find solutions that can support your work-life balance, such as flexible work arrangements or reduced work hours if possible.

9. Make time for self-reflection: Take the time to reflect on your work-life balance regularly. Assess how you are allocating your time and energy, and make adjustments as needed to ensure that you are prioritizing your personal well-being along with your work commitments. Regular self-reflection can help you stay mindful of your work-life balance and make necessary changes to maintain it.

10. Seek support: Don't be afraid to seek support from friends, family, or professional resources if you are struggling to achieve work-life balance. Surround yourself with a supportive network that can provide guidance, encouragement, and assistance when needed. Remember that achieving work-life balance is a continuous process, and it's okay to ask for help along the way.

Achieving work-life balance is an ongoing process that requires conscious effort, self-awareness, and commitment. It's important to recognize that work and personal life are not separate entities, but rather interconnected aspects of our lives that need to be integrated harmoniously. By defining your priorities, setting clear boundaries, planning and organizing your time, practicing self-care, learning to say no, delegating and prioritizing, unplugging from technology, communicating with your employer, making time for self-reflection, and seeking support when needed, you can create a fulfilling and balanced life that encompasses both work and personal pursuits.

Remember, work-life balance is unique to each individual, and what works for one person may not work for another. It's important to regularly assess and reassess your work-life balance and make adjustments as needed to ensure that it aligns with your personal values, priorities, and goals. By prioritizing your well-being and finding a healthy integration of work and personal life, you can lead a more fulfilling, balanced, and happy life. So, embrace the art of work-life balance and create a life that nourishes and fulfills you in all aspects!

CHAPTER 8: CULTIVATING MEANINGFUL RELATIONSHIPS

As humans, we are social beings who thrive on connection and meaningful relationships. Relationships play a crucial role in our lives, influencing our happiness, well-being, and overall quality of life. Whether it's our relationships with family, friends, romantic partners, or colleagues, cultivating meaningful relationships is essential for our emotional, mental, and physical health. In this chapter, we will explore the importance of meaningful relationships, how to cultivate them, and the benefits they bring to our lives.

The Importance of Meaningful Relationships

Meaningful relationships are those that are deep, authentic, and fulfilling. They go beyond superficial interactions and provide us with a sense of belonging, support, and purpose. These relationships are built on mutual trust, respect, and understanding, and they contribute significantly to our emotional and mental well-being.

Research has shown that people with strong social connections tend to live longer, healthier lives compared to those who are socially isolated. Meaningful relationships can have a positive impact on our mental health, reducing the risk of depression, anxiety, and other mental disorders. When we have meaningful relationships in our lives, we have a support system that we can rely on during challenging times, which can help us cope with stress and adversity.

In addition to improving our emotional and mental well-being, meaningful relationships also play a crucial role in our personal growth and development. They provide us with opportunities for self-reflection, learning, and growth. Meaningful relationships challenge us to become better versions of ourselves, as we learn from our interactions with others, gain new perspectives, and develop empathy and compassion.

Furthermore, meaningful relationships contribute to our sense of purpose and fulfillment in life. When we have people in our lives who truly care about us and whom we care about, we feel a sense of belonging and meaning. These relationships give us a reason to strive for personal growth, achieve our goals, and make a positive impact on the world.

Cultivating Meaningful Relationships

Building and maintaining meaningful relationships require effort, commitment, and genuine connection. It's not enough to simply have a large network of friends or acquaintances; it's the quality, not the quantity, of our relationships that matters. Here are some key principles for cultivating meaningful relationships:

Authenticity: Authenticity is the foundation of meaningful relationships. Being genuine and true to ourselves allows us to build trust and create a deeper connection with others. It's important to be honest, open, and vulnerable in our interactions with others, and to avoid pretending to be someone we're not. Authenticity fosters mutual understanding and respect, and it encourages others to be authentic in return.

Communication: Effective communication is essential for building meaningful relationships. It's important to actively listen to others, show empathy, and express ourselves honestly and respectfully. Good communication involves not only expressing our own thoughts and feelings but also understanding and validating the thoughts and feelings of others. Clear, open, and honest communication helps us to build trust, resolve conflicts, and deepen our connections with others.

Emotional Intelligence: Emotional intelligence is the ability to recognize, understand, and manage our own emotions and the emotions of others. It plays a crucial role in building meaningful relationships, as it allows us to empathize with others, regulate our emotions, and navigate social situations effectively. Developing emotional intelligence involves self-awareness, self-regulation, empathy, and social skills, and it contributes to healthy and meaningful relationships.

Shared Values and Interests: Meaningful relationships are often built on shared values and interests. When we have common beliefs, goals, or interests with others, it creates a sense of connection and belonging. Shared values and interests provide a strong foundation for building a meaningful relationship, as they give us common ground to bond over and create shared experiences.

Investing Time and Effort: Cultivating meaningful relationships requires time and effort. It's important to prioritize and invest in our relationships by spending quality time with our loved ones, showing appreciation, and being there for them during both good and bad times. It's not enough to simply have occasional interactions; consistent effort is needed to build and maintain deep connections with others.

Building Trust: Trust is a fundamental component of meaningful relationships. It takes time and consistency to build trust, and it can be easily broken if not nurtured. Trust is built through honesty, reliability, and keeping one's promises. Trust allows us to be vulnerable, share our thoughts and feelings, and rely on others for support. Building trust requires integrity, dependability, and being true to our word.

Boundaries: Setting healthy boundaries is essential in cultivating meaningful relationships. Boundaries help us establish a sense of self-respect and self-care, and they also allow others to understand and respect our needs and limitations. It's important to communicate our boundaries clearly and assertively, and to respect the boundaries of others as well. Boundaries provide a framework for healthy interactions and help prevent misunderstandings and conflicts.

Forgiveness and Conflict Resolution: No relationship is perfect, and conflicts are inevitable. However, how we handle conflicts and resolve them can greatly impact the quality of our relationships. Learning to forgive, let go of grudges, and resolve conflicts in a healthy and constructive manner is crucial for cultivating meaningful relationships. It involves effective communication, active listening, and finding solutions that are mutually beneficial. Conflict resolution skills contribute to stronger and more resilient relationships.

Empathy and Compassion: Empathy and compassion are essential qualities for cultivating meaningful relationships. Empathy is the ability to understand and share the feelings of others, while compassion is the willingness to show kindness, understanding, and support. Cultivating empathy and compassion involves being present, listening attentively, and showing empathy towards the experiences and emotions of others. It helps us build deeper connections with others and fosters a sense of care and concern.

Diversity and Inclusion: Meaningful relationships can also be cultivated by embracing diversity and practicing inclusivity. It's important to respect and appreciate the differences in others, including their cultural, ethnic, religious, and personal backgrounds. Embracing diversity promotes open-mindedness, understanding, and acceptance, and it enriches our relationships by bringing different perspectives and experiences to the table.

The Benefits of Meaningful Relationships

Cultivating meaningful relationships has numerous benefits for our overall well-being and quality of life. Here are some of the key benefits of having meaningful relationships:

1. Improved Mental Health: Meaningful relationships provide us with emotional support, reduce feelings of loneliness and isolation, and contribute to positive mental health. Studies have shown that people with strong social connections are less likely to experience depression, anxiety, and other mental health issues.

2. Increased Happiness: Meaningful relationships bring joy, laughter, and happiness into our lives. Having people who genuinely care about us and whom we care about creates a sense of belonging and purpose, which contributes to our overall happiness and well-being.

3. Enhanced Physical Health: Meaningful relationships also have a positive impact on our physical health. Research has shown that people with strong social connections tend to have better physical health outcomes, including lower rates of chronic diseases, better immune function, and faster recovery from illness or injury.

4. Greater Resilience: Meaningful relationships provide us with a support system during challenging times, which helps us cope with stress, adversity, and life's ups and downs. Having people who we can rely on and who provide us with emotional support and encouragement contributes to our resilience and ability to bounce back from difficult situations.

5. Personal Growth and Development: Meaningful relationships challenge us to grow and become better versions of ourselves. They provide opportunities for self-reflection, self-improvement, and personal growth. Through meaningful relationships, we learn to communicate effectively, resolve conflicts, practice empathy and compassion, and develop a greater understanding of ourselves and others. These experiences contribute to our personal development and growth as individuals.

6. Increased Life Satisfaction: Meaningful relationships are a key factor in overall life satisfaction. Having strong social connections and meaningful relationships brings fulfillment, purpose, and a sense of belonging, which contributes to our overall satisfaction with life. Meaningful relationships provide us with a sense of purpose and fulfillment, and they enrich our livesin numerous ways.

7. Support System: Meaningful relationships provide us with a support system that we can rely on during challenging times. Having people who genuinely care about us and whom we care about creates a sense of safety and security. We can lean on our loved ones for emotional support, encouragement, and guidance, which helps us navigate through difficult situations with resilience and strength.

8. Increased Happiness: Meaningful relationships bring joy, laughter, and happiness into our lives. Having people who genuinely care about us and whom we care about creates a sense of belonging and purpose, which contributes to our overall happiness and well-being.

9. Enhanced Social Skills: Cultivating meaningful relationships also helps us develop social skills that are essential in various aspects of life, such as communication, active listening, empathy, and conflict resolution. These social skills are not only important in our personal relationships but also in our professional and social interactions, contributing to our success and fulfillment in various areas of life.

10. Shared Experiences and Memories: Meaningful relationships create cherished memories and shared experiences that add richness and depth to our lives. The bonds we form with others through meaningful relationships are often based on shared experiences, adventures, and moments of laughter, joy, and celebration. These shared experiences create lasting memories that we can cherish throughout our lives, creating a sense of connection and belonging.

11. Opportunities for Giving and Receiving: Meaningful relationships also provide opportunities for giving and receiving. Through meaningful relationships, we can offer support, kindness, and compassion to others, and in turn, receive the same from our loved ones. Giving and receiving in relationships create a sense of reciprocity and mutual care, fostering a positive and nurturing environment where everyone feels valued and appreciated.

12. Enhanced Emotional Intelligence: Cultivating meaningful relationships also helps us develop emotional intelligence, which is the ability to recognize, understand, and manage our emotions and the emotions of others. Emotional intelligence plays a crucial role in building and maintaining meaningful relationships, as it helps us navigate through complex emotions, communicate effectively, and connect with others on a deeper level.

Tips for Cultivating Meaningful Relationships

Cultivating meaningful relationships is a lifelong journey that requires effort, intention, and commitment. Here are some tips for cultivating meaningful relationships in your life:

1. Prioritize and Invest in Relationships: Make a conscious effort to prioritize and invest in your relationships. Set aside dedicated time for your loved ones, show appreciation, and be present in the moment when you are with them. Invest in building and maintaining deep connections with others by consistently showing up, being reliable, and demonstrating that you genuinely care.

2. Practice Active Listening: Active listening is a key skill in cultivating meaningful relationships. Practice active listening by giving your full attention to the person you are talking to, maintaining eye contact, and avoiding distractions. Show genuine interest in what the other person is saying, and respond with empathy and understanding.

3. Show Appreciation and Gratitude: Express your appreciation and gratitude towards your loved ones. Show them that you value and cherish their presence in your life. Practice gratitude by acknowledging and being thankful for the positive aspects of your relationships, and express your appreciation towards the efforts, kindness, and love shown by others.

4. Practice Empathy and Compassion: Cultivating empathy and compassion towards others is essential in building meaningful relationships. Put yourself in the shoes of others, try to understand their perspective, and show compassion towards their emotions and experiences. Be kind, considerate, and supportive, and offer a helping hand when needed.

5. Communicate Openly and Honestly: Communication is the foundation of any healthy relationship. Cultivate open and honest communication with your loved ones. Express your thoughts, feelings, and concerns openly and respectfully, and encourage them to do the same. Practice active and effective communication skills, such as active listening, expressing yourself clearly, and resolving conflicts in a constructive manner.

6. Build Trust: Trust is a fundamental element of meaningful relationships. Build trust with your loved ones by being reliable, keeping your promises, and maintaining confidentiality. Be honest, transparent, and trustworthy in your actions and words.

Trust takes time to develop, but it is essential in cultivating meaningful and lasting relationships.

7. Foster Shared Activities and Hobbies: Shared activities and hobbies can create common ground and strengthen the bond between individuals. Engage in shared activities and hobbies with your loved ones, such as cooking together, hiking, playing music, or watching movies. These shared experiences can create cherished memories and deepen the connection between you and your loved ones.

8. Be Supportive in Good and Bad Times: Being supportive is crucial in meaningful relationships. Offer your support, encouragement, and care during both good and bad times. Celebrate the successes and joys of your loved ones, and be there to provide comfort and solace during their challenges and sorrows. Show that you genuinely care and are willing to be there for them in all circumstances.

9. Practice Forgiveness and Letting Go of Grudges: In any relationship, conflicts and misunderstandings can arise. It's essential to practice forgiveness and let go of grudges to cultivate meaningful relationships. Holding onto grudges and resentments can poison relationships and hinder their growth. Learn to forgive and move forward, and be willing to work through conflicts in a constructive manner.

10. Be Authentic and Genuine: Authenticity and genuineness are essential in cultivating meaningful relationships. Be yourself, and encourage others to be themselves as well. Avoid pretending to be someone you're not or pretending to agree with others for the sake of pleasing them. Authenticity allows for deeper connections and fosters genuine relationships built on trust and mutual respect.

11. Show Flexibility and Adaptability: Relationships are dynamic and require flexibility and adaptability. Be willing to adapt and adjust to the changing needs and dynamics of your relationships. Show flexibility in your expectations, plans, and responses. Be open to feedback and willing to work through challenges together with your loved ones.

12. Be Mindful of Quality Time: Quality time is crucial in cultivating meaningful relationships. Be mindful of the time you spend with your loved ones and make it a priority. Put away distractions, such as phones or other devices, and be fully present in the moment. Create opportunities for quality time, such as family dinners, date nights, or shared activities.

13. Practice Self-Care: Taking care of yourself is essential in cultivating meaningful relationships. When you take care of your physical, mental, and emotional well-being, you are better equipped to show up fully in your relationships. Make self-care a priority, and ensure you are nurturing yourself so that you can be present and engaged in your relationships.

14. Be Respectful and Considerate: Respect and consideration are crucial in any relationship. Treat others with kindness, respect their boundaries, and show consideration for their feelings and needs. Be mindful of your words and actions, and strive to create a respectful and inclusive environment in your relationships.

15. Be Patient and Understanding: Be patient and understanding with yourself and others. Relationships go through ups and downs, and it's important to be patient during challenging times. Practice understanding and empathy towards your loved ones, and be willing to work through difficulties together. Avoid rushing or pushing for immediate results, as meaningful relationships require nurturing and time to grow.

Cultivating meaningful relationships is a vital aspect of a fulfilling life. Meaningful relationships bring joy, support, and fulfillment to our lives, and they require intentional effort and care. By prioritizing communication, empathy, trust, authenticity, and self-care, you can foster meaningful connections with others that are built on a foundation of mutual respect, understanding, and support.

Remember that meaningful relationships are not about

perfection or having a large number of friends or acquaintances. It's about the quality of the relationships and the depth of the connection that matters. It's about being present, supportive, and genuine in your interactions with others. It's about creating a sense of belonging, trust, and mutual understanding that enriches your life and the lives of those around you.

So take the time to reflect on your relationships and consider how you can cultivate more meaning and depth in them. Practice the principles of effective communication, empathy, trust, authenticity, and self-care in your relationships, and be patient and understanding as you work towards building meaningful connections with others.

CHAPTER 9: THE SCIENCE OF HAPPINESS

As humans, we all seek happiness. It's the driving force behind many of our actions and decisions. We pursue relationships, careers, hobbies, and material possessions in the hopes of finding happiness. But what exactly is happiness? Is it just a fleeting emotion or something more profound and lasting? In recent years, scientists and researchers have been studying the science of happiness to uncover its mysteries and provide insights into how we can lead happier lives. Happiness, from a scientific perspective, is often defined as a state of well-being that encompasses a range of positive emotions, such as joy, contentment, and satisfaction. It's not just about momentary pleasures or external circumstances, but rather a deeper sense of fulfillment and life satisfaction. While happiness is subjective and can vary from person to person, researchers have identified several key factors that contribute to our overall sense of well-being.

One of the most significant findings in the science of happiness is that our genetics play a role in our happiness levels. Studies have shown that our genetic makeup can influence our predisposition to experience positive or negative emotions. Some people may have a genetic advantage when it comes to happiness, while others may have a genetic predisposition towards unhappiness. However, it's important to note that genetics are just one piece of the puzzle and that our environment and life circumstances also play a significant role in our happiness.

Another key factor in the science of happiness is our mindset and perspective. Researchers have found that our thoughts and beliefs about ourselves, others, and the world around us can greatly impact our happiness levels. Positive thoughts and an optimistic outlook can lead to increased happiness, while negative thoughts and a pessimistic mindset can contribute to unhappiness. Cultivating a positive mindset and practicing optimism through techniques such as gratitude, mindfulness, and positive affirmations can have a profound impact on our overall sense of well-being.

Social connections and relationships also play a crucial role in our happiness. Humans are social creatures, and studies have consistently shown that having meaningful connections with others is a fundamental human need. Positive relationships, such as close friendships, romantic partnerships, and supportive family ties, are associated with increased happiness and well-being. Spending quality time with loved ones, nurturing meaningful relationships, and building social support networks can contribute to our happiness levels and improve our overall well-being.

Another essential element of happiness is pursuing and achieving meaningful goals. Setting and working towards goals that align with our values and interests can provide a sense of purpose and fulfillment. Whether it's pursuing a career path that we are passionate about, engaging in a hobby or creative pursuit, or making progress towards a personal goal, having a sense of purpose and direction in our lives can contribute to our happiness.

It's important to set realistic and achievable goals that are meaningful to us and provide a sense of purpose and fulfillment.

Physical health also plays a significant role in our happiness. Studies have shown that regular exercise, adequate sleep, and a healthy diet can positively impact our mood and well-being. Exercise, in particular, has been found to release endorphins, which are known as the "feel-good" hormones, and can significantly improve our mood and overall happiness. Taking care of our physical health through regular exercise, healthy eating, and sufficient rest can contribute to our overall well-being and happiness.

Another crucial aspect of happiness is practicing self-compassion and self-care. Many of us tend to be overly critical of ourselves, setting high standards and expectations that can lead to self-doubt and unhappiness. Practicing self-compassion involves treating ourselves with the same kindness, understanding, and care that we would offer to a friend or loved one. It's about acknowledging our imperfections, being kind to ourselves, and practicing self-care to meet our emotional, mental, and physical needs. Practicing self, compassion and self-care can improve our self-esteem, self-worth, and overall happiness.

In addition to these factors, the science of happiness has also revealed the importance of practicing gratitude and mindfulness. Gratitude involves recognizing and appreciating the positive aspects of our lives, no matter how small they may seem. It's about shifting our focus from what we lack to what we have, and it has been shown to increase happiness and well-being. Mindfulness, on the other hand, involves being fully present in the moment without judgment, and it has been shown to reduce stress, increase resilience, and improve overall happiness. Incorporating gratitude and mindfulness practices into our daily lives can enhance our happiness and well-being.

Furthermore, giving back to others and engaging in acts of kindness and altruism can also contribute to our happiness.

Studies have shown that helping others and practicing kindness can increase our sense of purpose, connection with others, and overall happiness. Engaging in volunteer work, performing random acts of kindness, and practicing empathy and compassion towards others can not only make a positive impact on the lives of others but also improve our own well-being and happiness.

It's important to note that happiness is not a constant state, and it's normal to experience a range of emotions, including sadness, anger, and stress, as part of the human experience. However, by understanding the science of happiness and incorporating evidence-based practices into our lives, we can cultivate a happier and more fulfilling life.

Practical Tips for Cultivating Happiness:

Practice gratitude: Take time each day to reflect on the things you are grateful for. It could be as simple as a beautiful sunset, a kind word from a friend, or a delicious meal. Cultivating gratitude can shift your focus towards the positive aspects of your life and increase your overall happiness.

Nurture social connections: Spend quality time with loved ones, build meaningful relationships, and foster social support networks. Surrounding yourself with positive relationships can greatly impact your happiness and well-being.

Set meaningful goals: Identify and pursue goals that are aligned with your values and interests. Working towards meaningful goals can provide a sense of purpose and fulfillment, contributing to your overall happiness.

Take care of your physical health: Regular exercise, healthy eating, and sufficient rest are essential for your physical and mental well-being. Taking care of your body can positively impact your mood and overall happiness.

Practice self-compassion and self-care: Be kind to yourself, acknowledge your imperfections, and prioritize self-care. Treating yourself with compassion and taking care of your emotional, mental, and physical needs can enhance your self-esteem and happiness.

Practice mindfulness: Engage in mindfulness practices, such as meditation or deep breathing, to cultivate present-moment awareness without judgment. Mindfulness can reduce stress, increase resilience, and improve overall happiness.

Engage in acts of kindness and altruism: Give back to others, practice empathy, and perform acts of kindness. Helping others and practicing kindness can increase your sense of purpose and connection with others, contributing to your happiness.

Limit materialistic pursuits: While material possessions can bring temporary happiness, it's important to recognize that true happiness doesn't solely rely on external circumstances. Limit your focus on materialistic pursuits and instead prioritize experiences, relationships, and personal growth.

Cultivate a positive mindset: Practice optimism, positive affirmations, and reframing negative thoughts. Cultivating a positive mindset can significantly impact your happiness and well-being.

Seek professional help when needed: If you're struggling with persistent feelings of unhappiness, anxiety, or depression, don't hesitate to seek professional help. Therapy, counseling, or other forms of mental health support can provide you with tools and strategies to improve your happiness and well-being.

CHAPTER 10: EMBRACING CHANGE AND RESILIENCE

Change is an inevitable part of life. From small, everyday changes to significant life transitions, change is constantly occurring around us. However, many of us struggle with change and find it difficult to adapt to new situations. We may feel anxious, overwhelmed, or resistant to change, which can impact our well-being. In this chapter, we will explore the importance of embracing change and building resilience to navigate through life's challenges with grace and strength.

Change can take many forms, including changes in our personal lives, relationships, work, health, and the world around us. It may be planned or unexpected, welcomed or unwelcomed. Regardless of the type of change, it can evoke a range of emotions, such as fear, uncertainty, sadness, and excitement. It's normal to feel a mix of emotions when faced with change, as it disrupts our sense of familiarity and routine.

One of the key aspects of embracing change is to develop resilience, which is the ability to bounce back from challenges, adapt to new situations, and thrive despite difficulties. Resilience is not something we are born with, but rather a skill that can be developed and strengthened over time. It involves cultivating a positive mindset, building healthy coping mechanisms, and developing a flexible attitude towards change.

One of the fundamental elements of resilience is our mindset. Our mindset refers to our beliefs, attitudes, and perspectives about ourselves and the world around us. A growth mindset, which is the belief that our abilities and intelligence can be developed through effort and learning, is associated with higher resilience. When we have a growth mindset, we see challenges as opportunities for growth, rather than obstacles to overcome. We believe in our own ability to learn and adapt, which gives us the confidence to face and embrace change.

Another important aspect of resilience is building healthy coping mechanisms. Coping mechanisms are the strategies and behaviors we use to manage stress and difficult emotions. Healthy coping mechanisms can include seeking support from others, practicing self-care, engaging in physical activity, mindfulness, and other stress-reducing techniques, such as deep breathing or journaling. Developing a toolkit of healthy coping mechanisms can help us effectively manage the challenges that come with change and prevent us from falling into unhealthy habits or negative patterns of behavior.

Flexibility is also crucial in building resilience. Being able to adapt to new situations and navigate through uncertainty requires a flexible mindset. It's important to let go of rigid expectations and be open to new possibilities. Flexibility involves being willing to let go of the past, accept the present, and embrace the future with curiosity and an open mind. It's about finding creative solutions and being adaptable in the face of change.

Embracing change also involves managing our emotions. Change can trigger a range of emotions, and it's important to acknowledge and validate these emotions. It's okay to feel fear, sadness, or anxiety in the face of change. However, it's also important not to get stuck in these emotions and to actively work on managing them. Practicing self-compassion and self-care can be beneficial in managing our emotions and building resilience. Taking care of ourselves physically, mentally, and emotionally allows us to better cope with the challenges of change and navigate through them with grace and strength.

Another critical element of embracing change is to develop a support system. Having a network of supportive people who can provide encouragement, guidance, and perspective can greatly impact our ability to navigate through change. This can include family, friends, mentors, or professional support, such as therapists or coaches. Surrounding ourselves with positive influences and seeking support when needed can help us feel more resilient and capable of facing change.

It's also essential to remember that change can bring opportunities for growth and personal development. When we embrace change with an open mind and a positive attitude, we can discover new possibilities and learn valuable lessons about ourselves and the world around us. Change can challenge us to step out of our comfort zones, develop new skills, and broaden our perspectives. It can be an opportunity for self-discovery, self-improvement, and personal growth.

In addition, embracing change can lead to increased adaptability and resilience, which are essential life skills in today's fast-paced, ever-changing world. The ability to adapt to change and bounce back from challenges is crucial for success and well-being in various areas of our lives, including our personal relationships, careers, and overall mental health. Embracing change and building resilience can enhance our ability to cope with stress, problem-solve, and thrive in the face of adversity.

Practical strategies for embracing change and building resilience include:

Acceptance: Accept that change is a natural part of life and that it is inevitable. Acknowledge and validate your emotions, but also recognize that change is a part of the human experience.

Positive mindset: Cultivate a growth mindset, believing that challenges are opportunities for growth and learning. Embrace change as a chance to develop new skills, gain new perspectives, and expand your horizons.

Healthy coping mechanisms: Develop healthy coping mechanisms to manage stress and difficult emotions. This may include seeking support from others, practicing self-care, engaging in physical activity, mindfulness, and other stress-reducing techniques.

Flexibility: Be open to new possibilities and let go of rigid expectations. Be willing to adapt and find creative solutions in the face of change.

Self-compassion and self-care: Practice self-compassion and prioritize self-care. Take care of yourself physically, mentally, and emotionally to better cope with the challenges of change.

Support system: Build a support system of positive influences who can provide encouragement, guidance, and perspective during times of change.

Mindfulness: Practice mindfulness, which involves being present in the moment without judgment. Mindfulness can help you manage difficult emotions, reduce stress, and enhance your ability to adapt to change.

Focus on what you can control: Instead of dwelling on things you can't control, focus on what you can control. Identify the areas where you have influence and take action accordingly.

Learning and growth: View change as an opportunity for learning and personal growth. Reflect on the lessons you can learn from the experience and how it can contribute to your personal development.

In conclusion, embracing change and building resilience are essential skills for navigating through life's challenges. Change is inevitable, and it can evoke a range of emotions, but by cultivating a positive mindset, developing healthy coping mechanisms, practicing flexibility, and seeking support when needed, we can adapt to change and thrive in the face of adversity. Embracing change can lead to personal growth, increased adaptability, and resilience, which are crucial for success and well-being in today's ever-changing world. So, let us embrace change with an open mind, positive attitude, and a resilient spirit, and discover the opportunities it can bring into our lives.

CHAPTER 11: LIVING WITH PURPOSE AND PASSION

As the sun rose over the horizon, Sarah woke up with a renewed sense of energy and excitement. She had a deep sense of purpose that filled her heart and soul, propelling her forward in her journey of life. Sarah had discovered the power of living with purpose and passion, and it had transformed her life in ways she could have never imagined.

Living with purpose and passion was not something that came naturally to Sarah. She had spent many years feeling lost and unsure of her direction in life. She had followed the conventional path, pursuing a career that society deemed respectable, but it left her feeling unfulfilled and empty. It wasn't until she embarked on a journey of self-discovery that Sarah realized the importance of living with purpose and passion.

Sarah's journey began with deep introspection and soul-searching. She took the time to reflect on her values, her strengths, and her passions. She asked herself the tough questions: What truly mattered to her? What made her come alive? What did she want to contribute to the world? These questions forced her to confront her fears and break free from the societal expectations that had dictated her choices in the past.

Through this process of self-reflection, Sarah discovered her true purpose: to help others and make a positive impact on the world. She had always been passionate about social justice and environmental sustainability, but she had pushed those passions aside in pursuit of a "practical" career. Now, she realized that she could align her career with her purpose and make a meaningful difference in the world.

With newfound clarity and purpose, Sarah set out to make changes in her life. She made bold decisions, taking risks that she had previously been afraid to take. She left her unfulfilling job and pursued opportunities that aligned with her values and passions. She started volunteering for organizations that were making a difference in her community and took steps to reduce her own environmental footprint.

Living with purpose and passion brought a renewed sense of joy and fulfillment into Sarah's life. She found herself waking up with excitement and anticipation for the day ahead. Her work was no longer a mundane routine but a calling that filled her with a sense of purpose. She felt alive, energized, and motivated to make a positive impact on the world.

Sarah's newfound purpose and passion also had a ripple effect on other areas of her life. She became more authentic in her relationships, attracting like-minded people who shared her values and passions. She was no longer afraid to speak up for what she believed in, and she inspired others to join her in her mission to make the world a better place.

Living with purpose and passion also gave Sarah a sense of resilience and determination. She faced challenges and setbacks along the way, but her sense of purpose kept her going. She learned to persevere in the face of obstacles and setbacks, knowing that her work was bigger than herself. Her purpose gave her the strength and courage to keep pushing forward, even when the going got tough.

Sarah also learned the importance of self-care in living with purpose and passion. She realized that taking care of herself was not selfish but necessary for her to continue making a positive impact on the world. She made sure to prioritize self-care activities like exercise, mindfulness, and spending time in nature. She also surrounded herself with a supportive community of friends and mentors who encouraged and uplifted her on her journey.

Living with purpose and passion also brought a sense of balance and harmony into Sarah's life. She no longer felt like she was constantly chasing external achievements or societal expectations. Instead, she was guided by her inner compass and lived in alignment with her values and passions. This brought a sense of peace and contentment that she had never experienced before.

One of the most significant changes Sarah noticed was how her sense of time had shifted. Before, she used to count down the hours until the end of the workday, eagerly anticipating the weekends and holidays. But now, she found herself fully present and engaged in her work and activities, losing track of time because she was immersed in her purpose and passion. Time seemed to fly by, and she realized that living with purpose and passion had given her a newfound appreciation for the value of time.

Sarah also noticed that her creativity had flourished since she started living with purpose and passion. She was constantly coming up with new ideas and innovative solutions to the challenges she encountered in her work. Her mind was no longer constrained by limiting beliefs or societal expectations, but free to explore and create in alignment with her purpose. She felt a deep sense of fulfillment and joy as she tapped into her creative potential and made a difference in the world through her work.

Living with purpose and passion had also brought a deeper sense of connection to something greater than herself. Sarah felt a sense of interconnectedness with the world around her, realizing that her purpose was not isolated but part of a larger tapestry of humanity's collective efforts to make the world a better place. She found inspiration in the stories of other purpose-driven individuals who were also making a positive impact, and she felt a sense of camaraderie and solidarity with them.

Sarah's newfound purpose and passion also extended beyond her professional life. She found herself living with intention and mindfulness in all areas of her life, from her relationships to her hobbies to her daily habits. She made conscious choices that aligned with her purpose and brought her joy and fulfillment. She let go of things that no longer served her and made room for new experiences and opportunities that resonated with her authentic self.

Living with purpose and passion had also taught Sarah the importance of gratitude and appreciation. She learned to appreciate the small moments of joy and beauty in her life, whether it was a breathtaking sunset, a kind word from a friend, or a moment of connection with someone she was helping through her work. She realized that living with purpose and passion was not just about achieving big goals or making grand gestures, but about finding meaning and fulfillment in the everyday moments that made up her life.

Sarah also learned to embrace failure and setbacks as part of her journey. She understood that not everything would go according to plan, and that setbacks were opportunities for growth and learning. She learned to view failure as a stepping stone towards success, rather than a roadblock. Her sense of purpose and passion gave her the resilience and determination to bounce back from setbacks and keep moving forward with unwavering commitment.

Living with purpose and passion had a profound impact on Sarah's overall well-being. She felt happier, more fulfilled, and more content with her life. Her mental and emotional health improved as she aligned her life with her purpose and passions. She experienced a deeper sense of meaning and fulfillment, which translated into a greater sense of joy, peace, and overall life satisfaction.

Sarah's journey of living with purpose and passion also inspired those around her. Her friends and family noticed the positive changes in her and were inspired by her courage and determination to live a life aligned with her purpose. Sarah became a role model for others who were also seeking to live with purpose and passion, and she felt a deep sense of gratitude for the opportunity to inspire and impact the lives of others.

In conclusion, living with purpose and passion had transformed Sarah's life in profound ways. It had given her clarity, joy, resilience, and a deep sense of fulfillment. It had shifted her perspective on time, creativity, connection, gratitude, and failure. It had inspired her to live with intention and mindfulness in all areas of her life and had a positive impact on her overall well-being.

CHAPTER 12: CREATING A LASTING LEGACY

Legacy - a word that often brings to mind thoughts of great leaders, influential figures, and accomplished individuals who have left a lasting impact on the world. But legacy is not limited to the famous or the successful. It is something that each and every one of us has the power to create, regardless of our background or circumstances. In this chapter, we will explore the concept of creating a lasting legacy and how you can build a legacy that will endure for generations to come.

What is a Legacy?

At its core, a legacy is the mark or imprint that we leave behind in the world. It is the culmination of our actions, values, and beliefs that shape our impact on others and the world around us. A legacy can take many different forms, ranging from tangible accomplishments and contributions, such as inventions, works of art, or philanthropic efforts, to intangible legacies such as the way we inspire and influence others through our words, actions, and relationships.

One key aspect of a legacy is that it extends beyond our lifetime. It is the gift that keeps on giving, as it continues to influence and impact others long after we are gone. It is the mark that we leave on the world and the people we touch, even when we are no longer physically present. Creating a lasting legacy is about thinking beyond ourselves and considering how our actions today can shape the world for future generations.

Why is Creating a Lasting Legacy Important?

Creating a lasting legacy is important for several reasons. First and foremost, it is a way for us to make a meaningful contribution to the world and leave a positive impact that can outlast our lifetime. It gives us a sense of purpose and fulfillment, knowing that our actions have made a difference in the lives of others and have contributed to something greater than ourselves.

Secondly, creating a lasting legacy allows us to inspire and influence future generations. When we leave a positive legacy, we become role models for others to follow, and our actions can serve as a source of inspiration and motivation for others to make a difference in their own lives and in the lives of others. Legacy is a way to pass on our values, beliefs, and wisdom to future generations, creating a ripple effect that can continue to spread positive change in the world.

Lastly, creating a lasting legacy can also bring a sense of immortality. While our physical presence may not last forever, our legacy can continue to live on, carrying our name, values, and contributions forward into the future. It allows us to leave a lasting mark on the world and be remembered for generations to come.

Principles of Creating a Lasting Legacy

Creating a lasting legacy is not something that happens by accident. It requires intentional effort and planning. Here are some key principles to keep in mind as you strive to create a legacy that will endure:

Define your values and beliefs: Your legacy is an extension of your values and beliefs. It is important to take the time to reflect on what matters most to you and what principles you want to guide your actions. Consider what you want to be known for and what impact you want to make in the world. Clarifying your values and beliefs will provide a solid foundation for building your legacy.

Set meaningful goals: Having a clear vision of what you want to achieve is essential in creating a lasting legacy. Set meaningful goals that align with your values and beliefs, and strive to achieve them with passion and dedication. Your goals should be specific, measurable, achievable, relevant, and time-bound (SMART), and should reflect your desire to leave a positive impact on the world.

Take action with intention: Creating a lasting legacy requires taking action with intention. It is not enough to simply have good intentions; you must also take concrete steps to bring those intentions to life. Take deliberate and purposeful action towards your goals, consistently and persistently. Be proactive in identifying and seizing opportunities that align with your values and contribute to your legacy. Remember, it's not just about the quantity of your actions, but the quality and impact of those actions that truly matter in building a lasting legacy.

Cultivate meaningful relationships: Legacy is not just about what you achieve, but also how you impact others. Cultivate meaningful relationships with people around you - your family, friends, colleagues, and community. Be compassionate, empathetic, and supportive, and strive to make a positive difference in their lives. Share your knowledge, wisdom, and experiences with others, and be willing to learn from them as well. Building strong, authentic relationships can create a ripple effect that extends far beyond your lifetime and contributes to a lasting legacy of positive impact.

Leave a positive impact on your community and the world: A lasting legacy often involves making a positive impact on a larger scale - your community, society, or the world. Look for opportunities to contribute to causes or initiatives that align with your values and beliefs. This could involve volunteering your time, donating to charitable organizations, advocating for social change, or initiating your own projects to address societal or environmental issues. Your contributions to the greater good can have a far-reaching and lasting impact, leaving a legacy that embodies your commitment to making a positive difference in the world.

Continuously learn and grow: Creating a lasting legacy requires ongoing personal growth and development. Stay curious, open-minded, and willing to learn from new experiences and challenges. Embrace change and adapt to evolving circumstances. Invest in your own education and skill development to continually improve yourself and enhance your ability to contribute to your legacy. Remember, growth is a lifelong journey, and the more you learn and grow, the more impactful your legacy can become.

Lead with integrity and authenticity: Integrity and authenticity are crucial in building a lasting legacy. Be true to yourself, and let your actions align with your values and beliefs. Lead by example, and consistently demonstrate honesty, transparency, and accountability in your actions. Be genuine and authentic in your interactions with others, and strive to leave a positive impression through your integrity and authenticity. Your character and reputation are important components of your legacy, and they can have a lasting impact on how you are remembered.

Plan for the future: Creating a lasting legacy involves planning for the future, even beyond your lifetime. Consider estate planning, including a will and other legal documents, to ensure that your assets and contributions are managed according to your wishes. Think about how you want your legacy to be preserved and carried on by future generations. Consider mentoring or passing on your knowledge and skills to younger generations. Planning for the future allows you to have a deliberate and intentional approach to how your legacy will be sustained long after you are gone.

Embrace failure and setbacks as opportunities for growth: Legacy-building is not always smooth sailing. There will inevitably be challenges, failures, and setbacks along the way. Embrace these experiences as opportunities for growth and learning. Learn from your mistakes, adapt, and persevere. Don't let failure discourage or deter you from pursuing your vision of a lasting legacy. Instead, use it as a stepping stone towards greater resilience, wisdom, and determination in building a legacy that can endure.

Throughout history, there have been countless examples of individuals who have created lasting legacies that continue to inspire and impact others to this day. Let's take a look at a few examples:

Mahatma Gandhi: Gandhi's legacy as a leader of India's nonviolent independence movement is widely recognized and celebrated. His philosophy of Satyagraha, or nonviolent resistance, has inspired countless social movements around the world, and his unwavering commitment to peace, equality, and justice continues to inspire people to this day.

Nelson Mandela: Mandela's legacy as a leader in the fight against apartheid in South Africa and his unwavering pursuit of equality, justice, and reconciliation has left an indelible mark on history. His ability to forgive and seek reconciliation, even after spending 27 years in prison, has set an example for generations to come.

Mother Teresa: Mother Teresa's selfless dedication to serving the poor, sick, and marginalized in society has left a lasting legacy of compassion and humanitarianism. Her work with the Missionaries of Charity has inspired countless individuals to follow in her footsteps and make a difference in the lives of those in need.

Martin Luther King Jr.: King's tireless efforts in the civil rights movement in the United States, advocating for racial equality and social justice, have had a lasting impact on society. His iconic speeches, such as the "I Have a Dream" speech, continue to inspire people to fight for equality and justice for all.

Marie Curie: Curie's groundbreaking work in science, particularly in the field of radioactivity and her pioneering efforts in the advancement of women in science, has left a lasting legacy in the field of scientific research. Her achievements continue to inspire women and girls to pursue careers in STEM fields and make significant contributions to the world of science.

Creating a lasting legacy is about more than just leaving a mark on history; it's about making a positive difference in the lives of others and contributing to a better world. It requires intentional and purposeful action, guided by your values, beliefs, and vision for the future. By setting clear intentions, cultivating meaningful relationships, making a positive impact on your community and the world, continuously learning and growing, leading with integrity and authenticity, planning for the future, and embracing failure as an opportunity for growth, you can create a legacy that will endure long after you are gone.

Remember, your legacy is not solely determined by your achievements or possessions, but by the impact you have on others and the positive changes you bring to the world. It's never too early or too late to start building your legacy. Take action today and strive to create a lasting legacy that will inspire and impact generations to come. Your legacy is your gift to the world, so make it one that truly matters.

CONCLUSION : THRIVING IN HEALTH, WEALTH, AND WELL-BEING: YOUR JOURNEY TO SUCCESS

In conclusion, your journey to success is not just about achieving wealth and material possessions, but also about thriving in health and well-being. True success is holistic, encompassing all aspects of your life, including your physical, mental, emotional, and financial well-being. In this book, we have explored the interconnectedness of health, wealth, and well-being, and how they are essential elements of a fulfilling and prosperous life.

We discussed the importance of taking care of your physical health through proper nutrition, regular exercise, and self-care practices. A healthy body is the foundation for all other areas of your life, and investing in your health is an investment in your long-term success.

We also explored the significance of financial literacy and the importance of managing your finances wisely to create wealth and financial security. By adopting healthy financial habits, such as budgeting, saving, investing, and being mindful of your spending, you can build a solid financial foundation that can support your goals and aspirations.

Furthermore, we delved into the realm of well-being, which includes mental, emotional, and spiritual aspects of your life. We discussed the importance of cultivating a positive mindset, managing stress, nurturing meaningful relationships, and finding purpose and fulfillment in your life. Well-being is the glue that holds all areas of your life together, and prioritizing your mental, emotional, and spiritual health is crucial for overall success and happiness.

Throughout this book, we emphasized the importance of self-awareness, self-reflection, and continuous personal growth as key elements of your journey to success. Understanding your values, beliefs, strengths, and weaknesses, and aligning them with your goals and aspirations, can help you make informed decisions and create a fulfilling and purpose-driven life.

We also recognized that setbacks and failures are inevitable in life, but they can serve as valuable learning opportunities. Embracing failure as a stepping stone to success, rather than a roadblock, can help you develop resilience and perseverance, which are essential qualities for achieving long-term success.

In conclusion, thriving in health, wealth, and well-being is a lifelong journey that requires intentional and mindful efforts. It's about finding balance and harmony in all aspects of your life and creating a life that aligns with your values and brings you joy and fulfillment. By taking charge of your physical health, managing your finances wisely, nurturing your mental, emotional, and spiritual well-being, continuously growing and learning, and embracing failure as an opportunity for growth, you can create a successful and meaningful life.

Remember, success is not a destination, but a journey. It's up to you to define what success means to you and create a roadmap to achieve it. It's never too late to start, so take the lessons and insights from this book and embark on your journey to success, thriving in health, wealth, and well-being. May you find joy, fulfillment, and abundance in all areas of your life. Here's to your success!

www.ingramcontent.com/pod-product-compliance
Lightning Source LLC
Chambersburg PA
CBHW072339270726
48659CB00022B/2028